Your Story, Ahn's Story, and Our Stories

A Journal for Pre-Teen Girls

by

Susan Jo

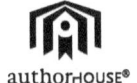

Bloomington, IN   Milton Keynes, UK

authorHOUSE®

AuthorHouse™
1663 Liberty Drive, Suite 200
Bloomington, IN 47403
www.authorhouse.com
Phone: 1-800-839-8640

AuthorHouse™ UK Ltd.
500 Avebury Boulevard
Central Milton Keynes, MK9 2BE
www.authorhouse.co.uk
Phone: 08001974150

First published by AuthorHouse   6/7/2007

ISBN: 978-1-4343-0769-9 (sc)

Printed in the United States of America
Bloomington, Indiana

This book is printed on acid-free paper.

Turn of the Century Spencerian calling card
Thank you to Grandma Kate and her friend Alma

Dedication

This book is dedicated to Dorothy Irene
and the music of her Pot Hole Creek.

Acknowledgements

Since this is a work of few words
appreciation must be brief:

To Autumn, Jackie, Jill, Jo, Leah,
Rachel and those who follow;

To Carole and Charla and the AzTechs
who began the journey with me;

To my husband, father, brothers, uncles,
son who offered respect along the way;

Thank you to Christine, Jenn, JoAnn,
Julie, Kathleen, Marquita, Miriam,
Pamela, and Sharon for the prompts.

And gratitude to the universe and the love.

Contents

Your Story

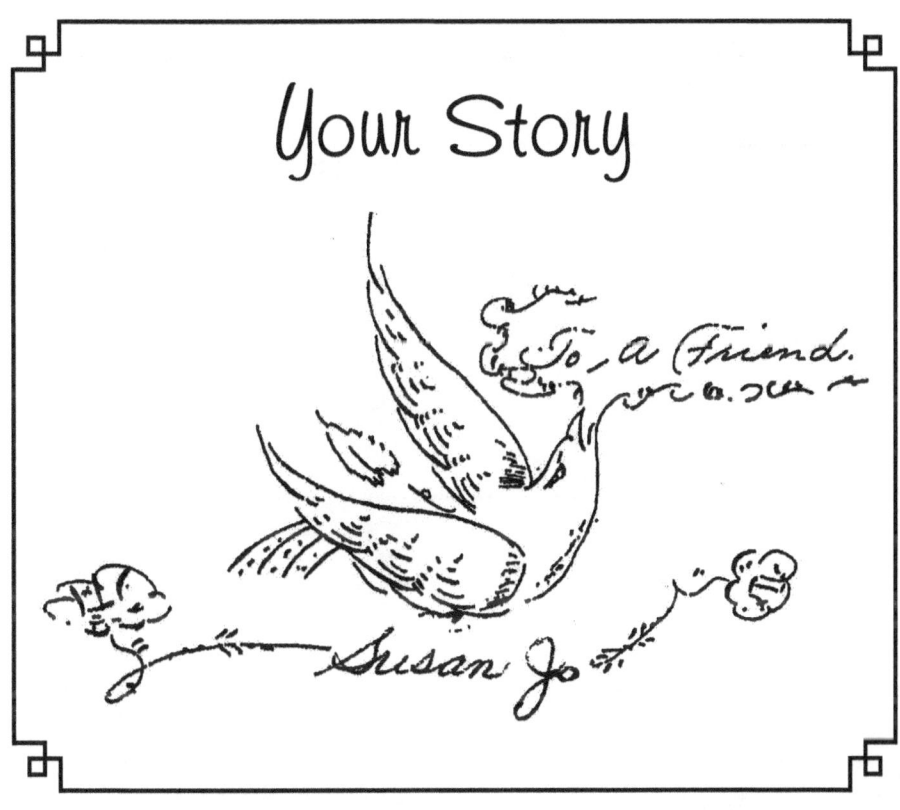

To A Friend.

Susan Jo

Introduction

This is a story about a girl, maybe a little older than you. She lived close to where you live, but she lived a long time ago. She lived before the pioneers, even before the Native Americans that were here when many of our ancestors came. While you read AHN'S STORY try to remember when you have walked in the woods in a park or near your town. Ahn had only the woods for her home, and she knew a lot about animals and plants and nature.

We live on a wonderful planet in a universe that allows for constant change. We have days for activity and nights for rest determined by Earth's rotation as it moves around the sun. We can tell the monthly changes by the way the moon looks to us in the night sky. Some men a long time ago chose for us to have 12 months. Actually, if we had thirteen months each one would have 28 days with one-day left over each year and one more left during leap year. Native Americans name thirteen moons each year in their traditions.

The angle the sun hits our Earth gives us different seasons. We need to learn about these rhythms that keep repeating themselves and how they effect our bodies and the plants and animals who share our planet. Today we are surrounded by artificial things that keep us from noticing the way our world changes. Electric lights for example keep us from watching the night sky change with the seasons. Many of us live in cities and are inside large buildings. Sometimes it is hard to know where the sun is in the sky. Our grandparents' grandmothers and grandfathers told the time of day with the sun; especially if they were farmers.

AHN'S STORY is also one story of growing up and becoming a woman. Adults give many different ideas about growing up and what it means. Ahn had few adults in her life to guide her, and yet she was able to accept the changes that came to her body and her life and find hope and joy.

If we know about the changes that happen in the universe, we will understand the changes in our own bodies. Women's bodies seem to be more tuned into the natural cycles of the Earth than men. Ahn noticed how the animals lived. She considered them part of her life. She noticed the trees and the moon cycles and the seasons.

Ahn also knew how important people who love us are. She realized their love could bring her peace and calm even when she was all by herself. Someone who loves you has given you AHN'S STORY to read. Sharing with this special person

in your life what it means to grow up and become a woman is an opportunity you have. After you read AHN'S STORY you may want to use the empty pages to write about changes you observe in the universe and changes that are happening to your body. You may have questions to write down about life. Questions are good.

Perhaps you will want to draw or paint or take some photographs to add to your writing. This might be a time in your life to write poetry, or a song. This may be your first journal or diary. One day you may want to read your own words from this time on your life journey. Many women find writing down their thoughts helps them grow. Changing and growing are things all human beings do throughout their lives—not just as children.

The pages on the left are yours. Years ago when paper was scarce, people would write from back to front, upside down or at an angle across already printed pages. You are invited to make this volume Your Story as well as Ahn's Story.

Ahn's Story

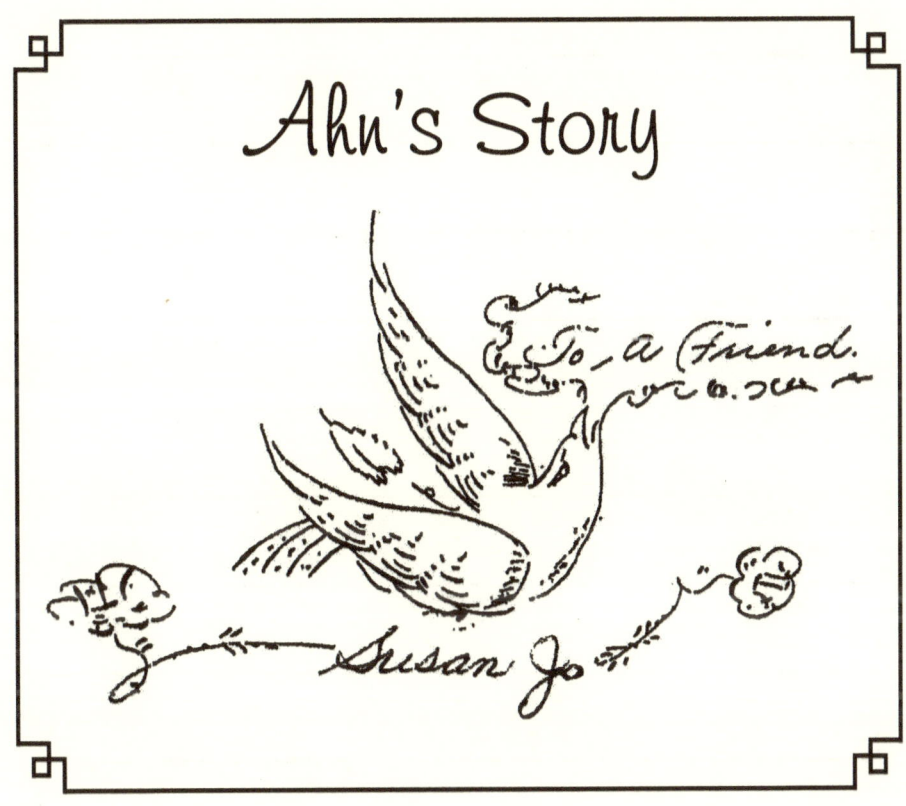

To A Friend.

Susan Jo

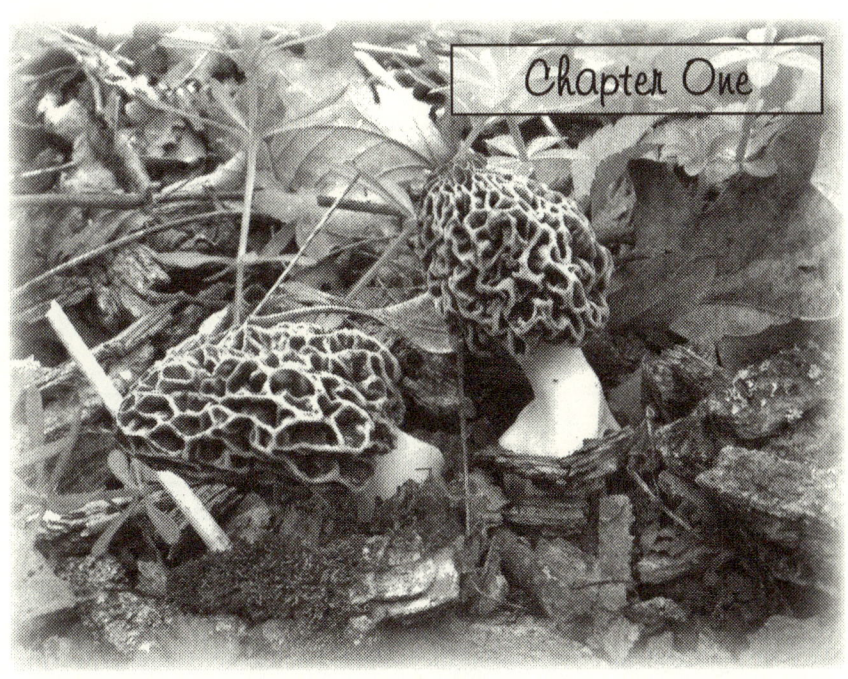

As she bent over the pain in her hips and back told her--only a few more stones today. Seeing the water begin to slow its course kept Ahn at the task. Ahn had found this special place surrounded by ferns, the beautiful hepatica and trillium. The constant water down the ravine had already carved out steps of basins in the limestone or loosened the softer materials revealing these fountain like bowls. It seemed an old place--one her ancestors must have known.

_____

_____

_____

_____

_____

_____

_____

_____

_____

_____

_____

_____

_____

_____

_____

She hesitated at first to change the sacred landscape. Still deep within came the sense that the sacred nature of this place was why she had been led here. Not a woman, not a child, every rock she had ceremoniously carried from the tumbled sides of the cliffwall had fit as if by plan. Now a reservoir of water was accumulating at the base of the small drop off.

She would come back tomorrow with her basket to collect moss for between the stones. The river was just below. Maybe she could catch the tiny fish and bring them to her bower.

The smell here was so filled with wet earth. Earth undercover of stonecrop, sedums and squirrel corn and delicate blossoms she didn't have a name for. Yet more than the beauty in her eyes, more than the cleanness in her nose was the water music in her ears. As the water left the sides of the limestone embankment and traveled from one basin down to another there was music. Each basin had its own clear tone.

Ahn knew it was time to leave when the light changed. The soft mosses that she laid her head on

to listen, just for a moment, now glowed gold from the sun's changing angle. She picked up the morels which filled her basket. Grandmother would never guess she had been creating a place for thinking about how she got here and who she was.

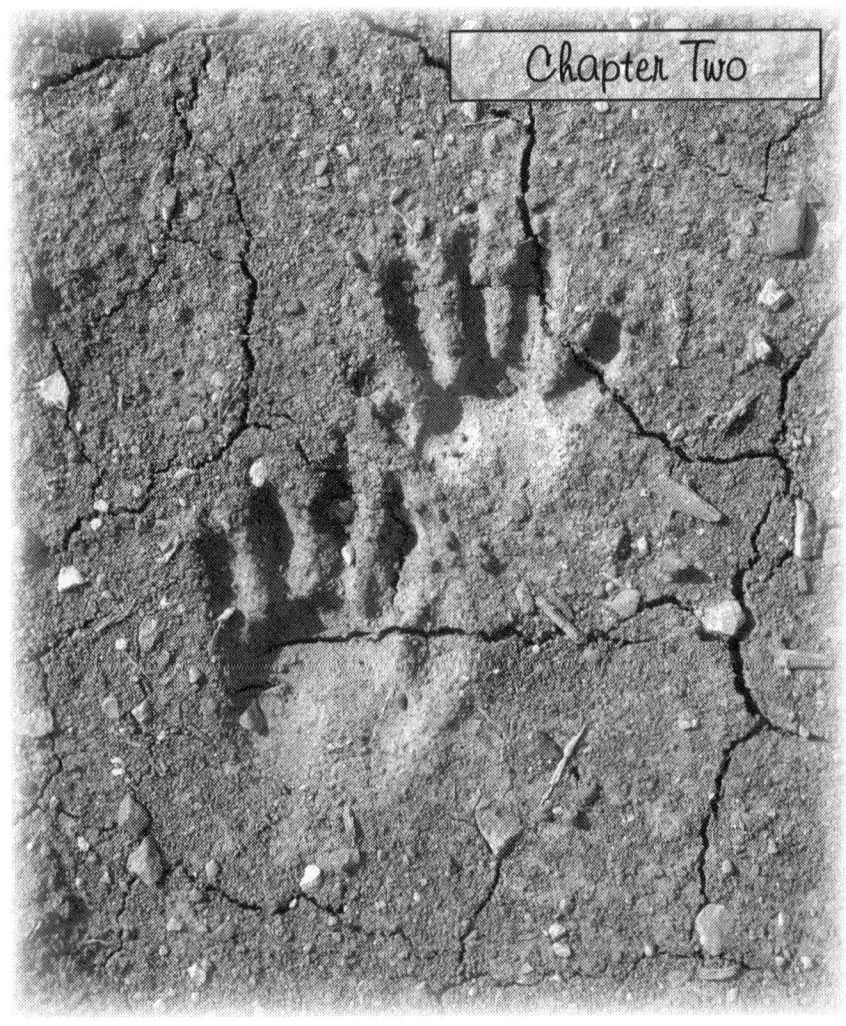

Chapter Two

There had been three sunrises before she could get back to her special place and the hard rain had pushed two of the smaller stones out of place. The wet leaves showed Ahn the water had risen above the top of her work. Now, it was well below it again. The

tiny footprints on the sandy place beside the stream made her think that the little creature with the mask might also have moved the stones. It may have been investigating.

Just now as she stood in the morning light, something from the bottom of the pool caught her eye. It was half of a shell. There were times Ahn watched at the river as the little fingers of the striped-tailed one cleaned out the soft remains from shells opened and discarded by the big grey bird that stands on one leg. And now the masked fellow had brought the shell up from the river to her pool. The shell made Ahn reach through her mind for ways to think about the sun drops of color.

She must bring her grandmother here. She had learned the names of plants they collected together. Some plants they dried to use later. Some they ate fresh. The wild ginger root, the asparagus, the ginseng were familiar names. Ahn wondered what the creatures' names were besides ones she made up for them. Ahn also needed words for the beauty and

color she saw at her special place. Did Grandmother think about these things that inside gave Ahn such a fullness? What she saw filled her eyes. She also breathed, listened, touched and tasted this place. And she needed more words. She needed to share what welled up in her and brought bubbles of laughter and humming breaths while she sat very still here.

The moss she gathered while walking to her special place helped stop the dribbles between the rocks. The darkness on her stones began moving up toward the top. Ahn found five more stones to finish her work. She stopped to admire what had happened here. Her work was an outer way of showing how she felt inside. Before leaving this time she thought about all of the small creatures that might come to this special place. The fish with legs and spots like sunshine and the tiny, tiny hopping one. She wanted to hide and watch. She felt connected to them, to the stones she had placed, to the light, to the colors of the broken shell.

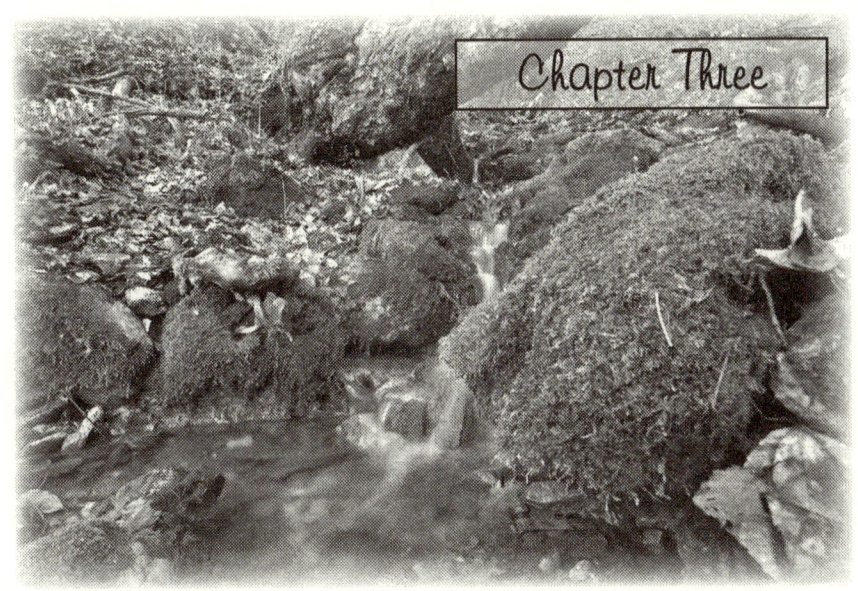

Chapter Three

Thankfully, Ahn was able to come back two more days to her place of thinking before she and her grandmother must follow the uncles again. Both times the sun was coming through the sweet new leaves above. She knew that some of the tiny buds tasted good, and that the deer knew this. By the time she saw this place again it would be without the sun. It would be under a canopy. The trees here were large. They stood together. The leaves opened and grew on these gigantic trees into a roof. Coming together at the top, the leaves

changed from a color that was full of light to one that darkened and deepened. Her family always left to go to an open place when the sun got higher in the sky. Grandmother said there were times of sickness if one stayed in the cool shadowed places. There were so many things to eat here, but also so many things that bit and made Ahn want to rub her skin off.

Ahn looked at each stone she had moved. They did not look out of place, but as if they belonged. Water came softly over the top now, and the moss seemed to be thriving. She wondered what it would be like as the seasons changed. The stones themselves now had colors since they stayed wet. She picked up a small worn rock, smooth and held it against her face. Then she wedged it into a hole in her clothing that was made of skin from the beautiful deer. She wanted to take something with her, so her mind would remember each detail. She would wet the stone to see the colors. Into the rock she placed everything before her. If she didn't

see this place soon, the rock's smooth, cool touch against her cheek would help her find the place in her mind.

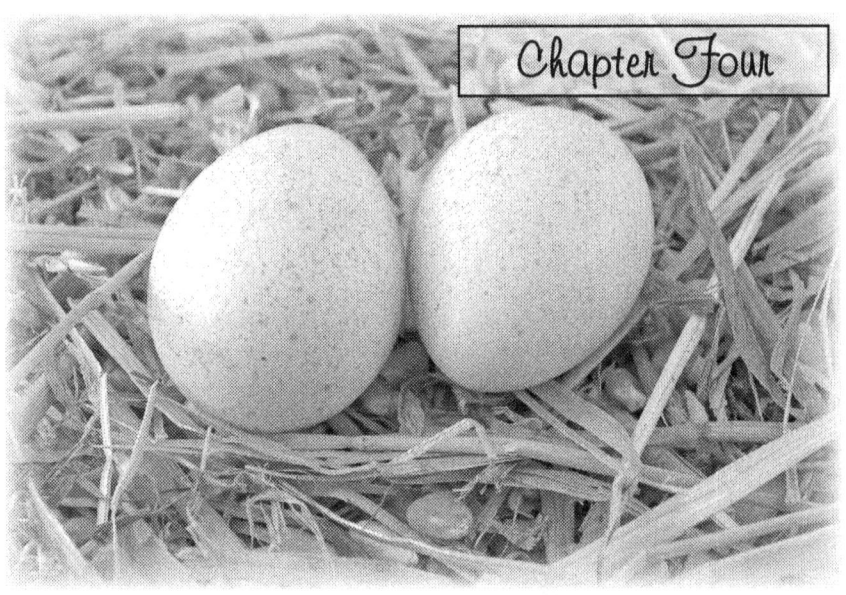

Chapter Four

Ahn was surprised to find her family gone.
She came from the quiet place ready to help her
grandmother gather their robes. All else could be
returned to the forest. But these things had been
done. Leaves were scattered back over their fire pit.
There was no sign of Grandmother, the two uncles
or where they had stayed these several months.

Ahn felt strange. Each day in her life that she
could remember was different than the day before.
She knew that change was to be expected. It kept
her mind sharp as they moved from place to place.

Home did not mean a certain spot, her whole world was her home. Sometimes the shelter was a cave; sometimes pine trees provided a soft bed of needles. But home had always meant the same people.

She reached for the smooth rock and pulled it loose. She wanted to stay here. Her thoughts surprised her. This was a new feeling. She had followed Grandmother and the uncles without ever thinking before. But now she had a stake in where she was. She would have to pay attention to where she was and where she would go. Being mindful of her surroundings came as a good feeling. She knew she would come back here even without the others. She would remember.

The white trees now became her landmarks. Grandmother called them sycamores and boiled their bark sometimes to rub on their skin. Instinctively, she knew these trees followed the river just as she must. On hot sun-filled days she walked the river's cool center. On rainy, stormy days she found the largest white trees, hollowed out by age and used

_____

_____

_____

_____

_____

_____

_____

_____

_____

_____

_____

_____

_____

_____

_____

them as her place of rest. The river's rise sometimes sent her higher up into the giant trees' arms. Ahn took side trips to gather and eat berries or to dig for tubers. But in the corner of her vision were always the large white river trees.

The night sky had gone around from a new moon to a full face before Ahn caught up with the others. The river was now wider and swifter. One had to stay on the bank now. She had seen the smoke two days before she saw them. There was no sign of the uncles, but grandmother was cooking meat over the fire. Ahn's hunger made her steps go faster. Ahn was curious as to why they had left her. Fear was unknown to her; acceptance was easier.

Grandmother smiled a welcome as though she was confident Ahn would find them. The uncles had thought her old enough to find her own way Grandmother said. Both uncles returned with turkey eggs. They would make this a celebration. For now Ahn was feeling warm inside to be with her family, knowing they were pleased with her

accomplishment. And yet the smooth rock was still hers. She would remember how to return to her quiet place.

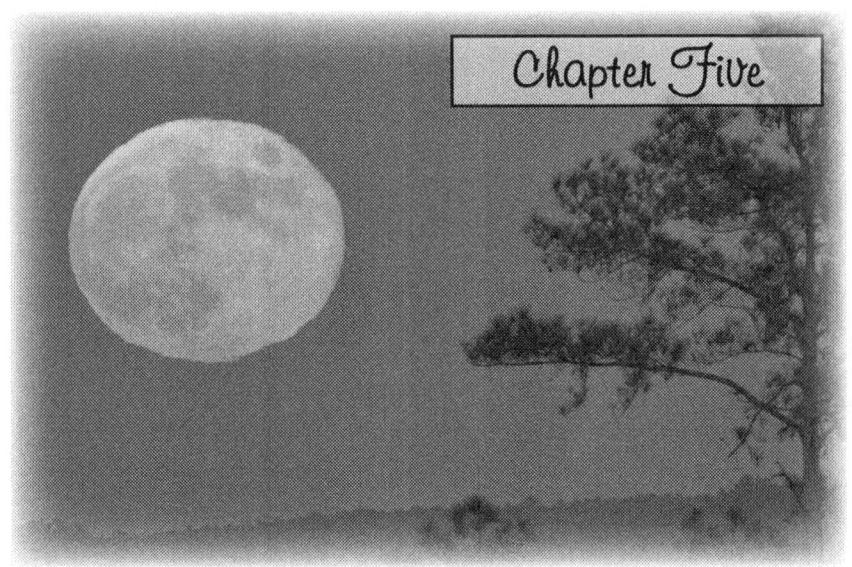

Chapter Five

Ahn awoke suddenly. There was a pain and the dream clear and present with her. She had a feeling in her groin that made her want to curl in on herself. Strangely, there was a stickiness between her legs. She felt she knew her body well. Her swelling breasts and darkened nipples were a part of her now as were her longer legs. The dream started to slip away and then it came back as a fully colored scene.

She was in the pool of her creation that was made in the Spring. A sleek doe was looking at her at eye level. Their gaze held long enough for Ahn to be filled with the peace offered to her by the beautiful female

being. Ahn knew now why her uncles had left her. She had seen the blood of moons on animals in the woods when they were ready to be together. It was a powerful sign.

She sensed, too, the danger that came with this issuance. Her dream deer had faded. She looked up to see a full, round moon which was large and red even as it climbed the night sky. This had always meant a seasonal change for Ahn--this sky filling moon. Cold nights were soon to be.

Ahn tried to go back to sleep, but found herself enjoying a new sensation. Created by rocking her legs across each other the feeling rose directly to her breasts. Her breaths came mostly as those that would put out the flame of a small twig in the fire. As she breathed in, a slow tingling moved up her body and waited to be shared. A pleasant sleep returned.

Sunlight held her face warm. Sluggishly Ahn shook her sleep away and found herself alone again. She was covered by a warm fur robe. Her first waking sense included the smell of blood. This was not unfamiliar;

most living creatures that were eaten gave their blood, their life force. Ahn knew, however, that this was different. This smell came from her own loins. The blood lost pooled thickly in the dust underneath her. There was no more time to enjoy strange new rumblings in her body. Urgency came to her to keep the smell separate from herself. Too many creatures of the earth used blood as an attractor.

This time on finding herself alone she took her time. She bathed close to the shore of the big river. She would need the robe left by her uncles and grandmother. She rolled it carefully, pushing it under a heavy rock. She knew right then a way to hold the blood. Clean green mosses folded over themselves could be placed high and held by the strong muscles at the top of her legs. When the mosses became heavy and dropped away Ahn buried them. She'd been taught to do this whenever the food she ate came back out of her body. Ahn knew other animals claimed their territory by leaving excrement and even evidences of blood on top of the ground. The dung

beetles and other orange and black bugs cleaned this and the dead animals up. Yet it seemed important to her to use the clean earth to cover all she left behind. All this instruction came from the voice inside her. Grandmother had never spoken of any of this, but Ahn always tried to be observant.

Though she was wishing to be back at her special place, she didn't try and catch up with the others. This was her time.

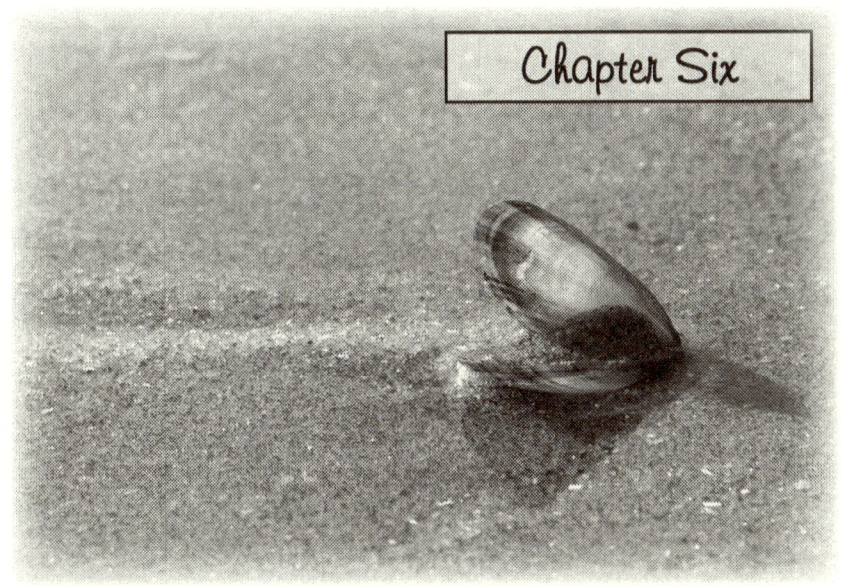

Chapter Six

Here by the White River she watched the water birds with new thoughts. Some she knew were feeling seasonal yearnings to leave for another place, too. Why had she never considered those that fly before, Ahn asked herself? She saw beauty never noticed in their changing hues that varied with movement and with the sun and water. The only work was to care for herself. Grandmother had left a cache of good acorns from the rounded leaved trees and a rough rock nearby for grinding. She competed for berries with more of the flying ones. These were plump and

their breasts colored like the jewel weed. She heard their songs in a new way. They did not swim. These she remembered were not heard during the colder months.

The large grey and white ones her uncles had caught and cooked before were noisy coming and going along the river's edge. Ahn could see them a long way as they rose together and formed a flying arrow in the sky.

Eating as always required the most thought. The solitary glide of the fisherman bird caught Ahn's eye. She was able to grab the fish he had speared as it fell from his grasp. He cut loose on her with a loud series of squawks, but soon dove again and held onto his catch.

Ahn watched the tall one standing on one leg and this time she cleaned up the mussel fragments. She watched a swimming and flying one feeding its young high in the trees. The young, fully feathered fell right into the river from their nest and swam with their parents. Their rainbow colors caught light

as if by magic and a headdress gave them a look of importance.

Raw fish was her lot without her uncles and Grandmother who supplied the fire. Her energy began to return after three days by herself. She wrapped the robe around herself, erased any sign of her stay by the river, and began to go the way her family would have gone.

Ahn wanted to ask her grandmother the most important question she could ask. It had never come to her before, but now she knew. She was female like Grandmother though as far as she knew, Grandmother never had the flow of blood. But in her heart Ahn knew to have a grandmother was to have a mother. Once she had cared for tiny foxes whose mother had been killed. She watched, she knew. But to put into words that question, "Where is my mother?" and the one that came with it, "Will I be a mother?" was almost impossible. She knew the uncles called Grandmother the same as she; but that they were different. They only used the term grandmother in

reference to her. "Your grandmother wants this or that." "Go take this to your grandmother." She had accepted all of this until now. Now that she had been left behind twice, now that she could make her way on her own, now that her body had made this major change, she needed to know more.

Her pace sped up. Only Grandmother would know the answers she sought. There had been talk of ancestors, but no talk of mothers. The question had been forming under the surface of her life for as long as she could remember. Thus, it came out specific and accompanied by other questions even though it was new and never asked before. Where is my mother? How did I get here? How can I be a mother?

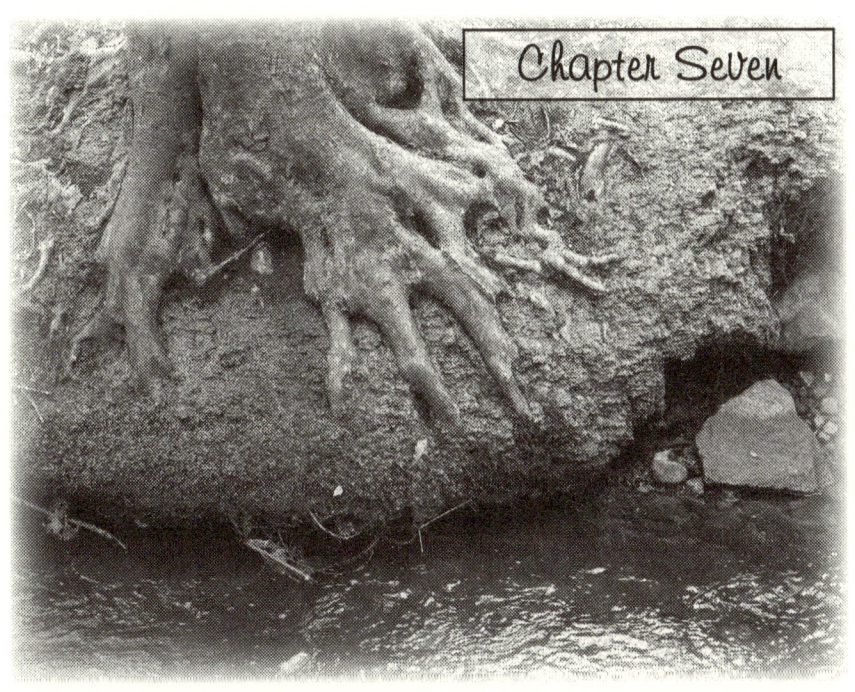

Chapter Seven

For once Ahn didn't notice her world as she traveled. She knew the way back along the waterway to the cliffs without thinking. Colder nights meant caves.

Ahn also knew the uncles were made different from her. This was all right and had never been anything to consider before. She had seen the buffalo who let their water go in different ways.

Confusion clouded Ahn's thinking. This felt as new to her to be thinking of these things as the new

sensations in her body. The restlessness of her being made her as tired as the trek. Usually sure-footed, she found her lack of concentration emphasized when she missed seeing roots and stones and fell hard. Was this awkwardness part of the changes in her body? The rock she carried from her special place pushed against her skin as she picked herself up from her last fall. To be back at her special place now meant going back to a time in her life without disturbing questions.

Smoke ahead and steeper climbing found grandmother and one of the uncles waiting for her. Ahn knew she had been in this cave another time. Its familiarity helped her uneasiness just as grandmother's welcoming arms.

Talking was not encouraged. After Ahn was given food and a place was made for her to sleep in the warmth of the cave, she and Grandmother were alone. Now was the time. "Grandmother", Ahn began respectfully, "I am growing tall, I am

becoming as I am to be. My body is like the animals. Will I be a mother soon?"

"No, Ahn," Grandmother responded. "It takes more than your body changing. Sometimes becoming a mother means you will find another family. Your uncle has gone to try and find someone for you and someone for himself. We cannot go on as a family without others. It may mean you will go and I will have a new daughter to help me. We will see."

The question of her own mother's presence lay ready to speak, but Grandmother turned her back to Ahn and slept. Ahn was left with new ideas. But the rock she rubbed against her cheek again, gave her peace, and she slept well from her long walk.

Ahn awoke before sunrise in the middle of deep thought. Her coming of age was like the roots and rocks she kept catching her feet upon. Suddenly, there were outside-expectations of how things would be in her life. She was expected to find her way alone. She was expected to protect herself as she journeyed into new areas. Now she was to have

someone else in her life or go with someone else to another family. And this would mysteriously lead to becoming a mother when she had never known a mother.

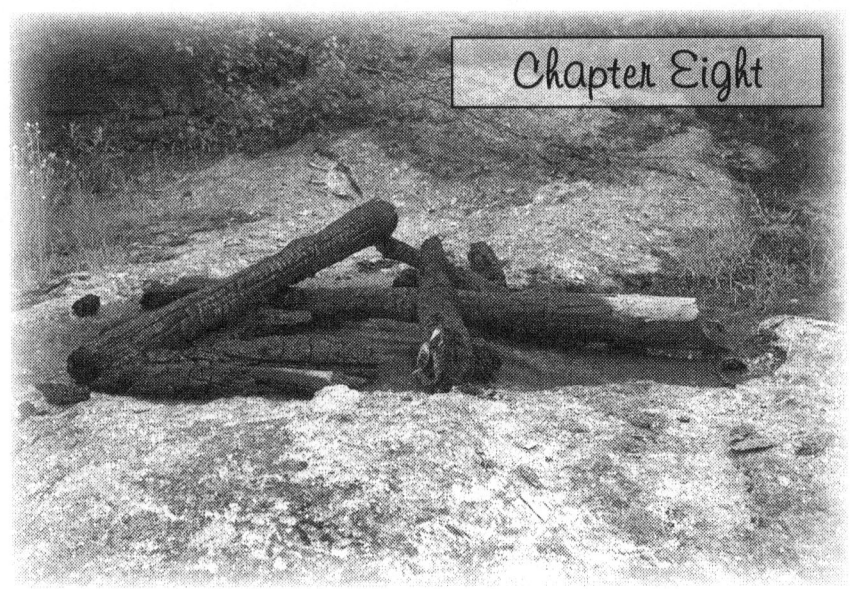

Chapter Eight

Ahn didn't ever ask the question. Her grandmother was suddenly very ill. Ahn sat with her every day in the cave. When the uncle finally came back, he brought with him new things. He shared some meat that was salted and dried, some flat white pieces that could be eaten and something he called beads that had the colors of light. Ahn loved these magic rocks with holes in them threaded on grass like strings.

Grandmother could not eat unless they put the small cakes in water. Soon Grandmother didn't want even that. Ahn tried to find soft berries for her. This

would be a long winter. What grandmother had done, Ahn must now do. The uncles went rock hunting and spent time making tools for hunting. Animals and birds they brought back were Ahn's to prepare. Keeping the fire going at the front of the cave was Ahn's job during the day. Grandmother did not talk any more; she grew very thin.

The only time Ahn had to herself was the three days when the moon was full and her blood flowed. There was a room in the cave off by itself. There was very little light here but a small stream she could wash in. The uncles made it clear she was to be by herself, and they would tend grandmother. One afternoon Ahn used some charcoal from the fire and drew pictures on the wall of her room. She wanted to remember the doe in her dream and somehow was able to draw it running. This seclusion was strange, but it gave Ahn a chance to rest and enjoy her body. The sandy bottom of the cave felt good on her skin and she rubbed it all over. Again, she buried the blood. One morning she wondered if she could use the blood on

the wall. Once it dried completely the smell would be gone. She took a stick and drew a bird, and she drew herself alone.

Once again energy renewed itself after three days, and she felt her grandmother needed her. The uncles had gone out, and Grandmother put her hand in Ahn's and gave a fragile squeeze. The grandmother hoarsely whispered, "You are a woman, Ahn, it is not easy. You are with the whole world. Cherish Ahn, cherish the world." That was all. Grandmother spoke no more. She closed her eyes, and two days later she quit bringing breath into her body.

Ahn cried as did the uncles. They lit a fire and sang a sad, sad song of goodbye that showed their pain. The uncles gently carried Grandmother's body up into one of the large, white, trees far from the cave. Here, the big birds would find it and pick the bones clean. They used grasses to tie the body to the tree. Then the three moved back to the cave.

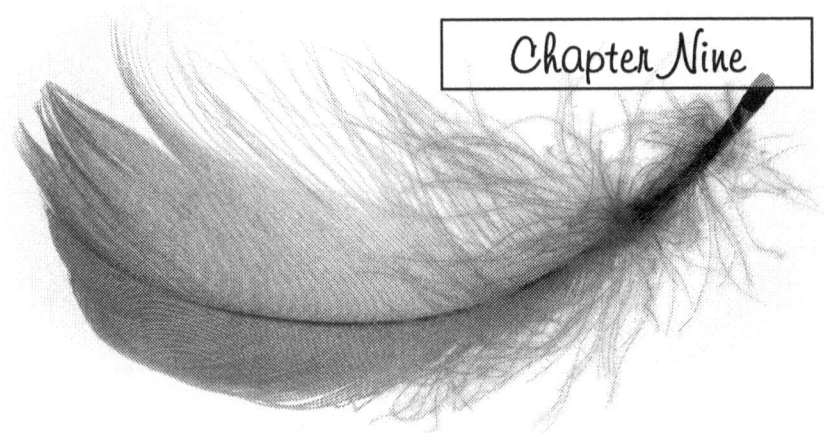

Chapter Nine

Ahn went back to work finding herself very alone much of the time. The pain inside hit her every morning she awoke without Grandmother. The uncles, too, grieved. It was a time of not knowing. The dark winter days made crying even easier for Ahn. All of the dark hours were spent sleeping. Snow outside made it harder for Ahn's uncles to find food. The meat that was salted was chewed and chewed. Ahn helped by finding acorns under the snow, some hidden by the bushy tail ones. Some were bitter even after grinding them, but Ahn remembered winter wasn't forever. She thought about the warmth of Grandmother's body that had held her all the winters before. She thought

of her first memory of Grandmother holding her and singing over and over her name. Was it her name or just the sound Grandmother made when she rocked her back and forth as a child? Her name was like the sound that came from Ahn now as she rocked herself back and forth and the tears ran down her cheeks.

"Cherish the world, cherish Ahn," Grandmother had said. Now her pictures were made in the sand of her private room and erased each time. The sadness held her close.

Before they were ready to leave the cave after the snow had gone, Ahn went to see Grandmother's body. A few bones that had not fallen into the river were all that was left and two colored beads that the uncle had put near the body. A perfect feather lay across the smallest bone. It was a darkish green with a yellow shaft. Ahn held the shaft in her mouth while she fashioned a pouch from a piece of her robe, using grass to tie it. She knew Grandmother would not need the bone now that her breath had gone somewhere else. Sometimes Ahn felt grandmother's breath very close.

She also decided to put the beads of color and light and her rock from the special place into the pouch. For a time she sat very still holding the rock and holding the bone and breathed slowly in and out. The feather vibrated her lips as if it were alive; she remembered that Grandmother was gone when she no longer breathed in the life force. Ahn brought in the life force evenly and slowly and let it out in little breaths. Peace became part of her. Glimpses of Grandmother at Ahn's special place walked through her mind. Someday she would take Grandmother's bone there.

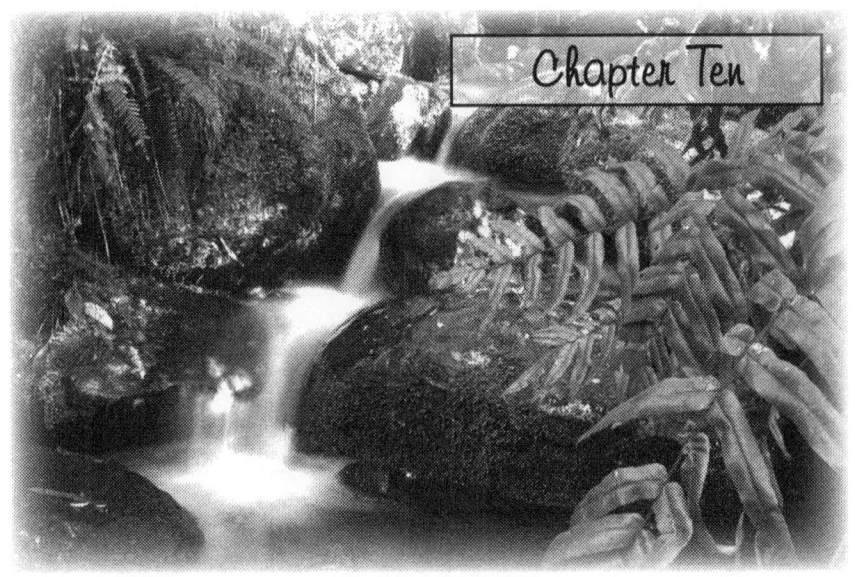

Chapter Ten

The uncles started off a new way. It was before there were any spring flowers, but the mosses were green and fresh and there were new green plants under the leaves that had fallen before the snow.

The path they followed was not one of their making. Ahn grew surprised to see other footprints on this path. The load she now carried of robes was bigger with Grandmother gone. When her time alone came and the blood flowed, she had to keep moving. Although the uncles did not wait on her, the length of their daily treks lessened. She stayed to herself when they stopped and walked behind a ways. They

didn't cook on those days. She missed the time of thinking, but the walking made the three days easier for her body. She was getting stronger, growing even more.

She asked one of the uncles where they were going. He smiled and said, "To the big world, You will be surprised." Ahn's only world had been the one her Grandmother had told her to cherish. Now what must she learn to cherish. It was from a new moon to another new moon to get there. There were hints as they got closer. Small family groups like theirs had camps along the way. Ahn was so amazed to see other persons and other women like her. Ahn felt the need to know another woman. Grandmother's death left her more than alone. Ahn did not have the word friend in her mind. She tried to come up with an idea that included how there could be other women in her life. She was shy, and the uncles did not stop as they passed these camps. Once she made eye contact with a girl younger than herself, and the girl smiled. Ahn cherished this smile in her heart and smiled back.

When they stopped to camp for the evening, she cooked if there was something the uncles caught during the day or a fish caught after they arrived. They were never far from a river. But now the river was so wide and deep, Ahn didn't see how they could ever get across. Ahn saw men like her uncles in boats on this river. She imagined herself floating down the river. She had hung her pouch around her neck. Somehow when she took out her rock that came from her peaceful place, other places became places of peace for her. She sensed that her life was going to be different from this point on. She could not control what would happen next. But in her peaceful heart, she prepared herself for more change. She yielded herself to the voice inside of her that came first from loving her grandmother. This same voice inside her heart had brought her a fullness at the special place she had created. Even with Grandmother gone, this presence inside her heart made thoughts of Grandmother come and fill Ahn with sadness but also with joy.

Concluding Comments

To a Friend.

Susan Jo

Now you have read about Ahn and perhaps you want to know more about her. So do I, but right now there is no more of the story for me to write. One option you and your mother/mentor could explore is writing about what happens to Ahn yourself. She emerges from her forest home and steps into…

Human beings are very resilient. People move from one culture, one bio-region to another and create very satisfying lives. In my mind I had glimpses of Ahn finding a friend, a girl or a boy who would share his/her family with her. I even pictured the friend's mother becoming like a mother to Ahn. I could see in my mind's eye Ahn becoming a mother herself in a more complicated world than she grew up in. This is kind of how each woman's life progresses. Complexity often increases as we celebrate each birthday. If we learn what is really important about living as a human being, as a woman-- often we can keep our lives more simple and calm.

Women are so fortunate; our bodies themselves help us remember the important things:

"Though there is certainly a place for decisiveness and action, there is also a place for patience. Have you learned when to wait?

Wait for the sunrise…there will be another day.

Wait for guidance… learn to be still.

Wait for wisdom…it will come with experience.

Wait for growth…it happens in the fullness of time.

Wait and be contented…it is a secret to inner peace.

There is a time to act, but there is also a time to wait. Learn how to tell what time it is, for great things can happen for those who learn to wait." Ralph Waldo Emerson said it well: "Adopt the pace of nature; her secret is patience." From <u>www.lifesupportsystem.com</u> Steve Goodier

Our Stories

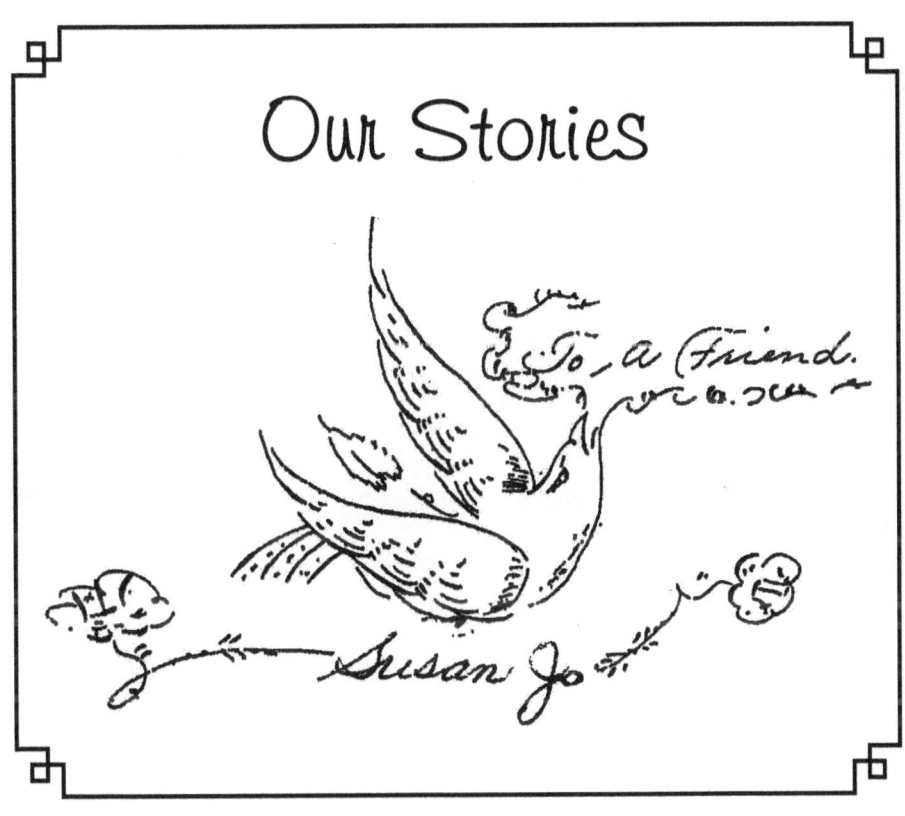

To A Friend.

Susan Jo

Life changes over several years called forth a story about a young girl in a hunter-gatherer society from my heart. The story takes place in Southern Indiana where I live. Two forces seemed to be at work as this final product developed:

Primary was my desire to help young people to find their center in nature. My parents nurtured this in me and as a mother I encouraged love of all of nature's forces and creatures as a focus of my child rearing. The power of meditation, the practice of mindfulness, the concept of eldering all came into play as the story unfolded. My awareness of Thomas Berry's and Brian Swimme's <u>The Universe Story</u> also culminated in AHN'S STORY.

Secondarily, the age and sex of the main character in the story brought with it the natural experience of her first mense. I was not up to date on children's literature, and I expected to find several , more polished examples of fiction which explored a girl becoming a woman in the physical sense as well as emotionally and mentally. I thought my story would be unique only in its ties to the natural world and the pre-historic time frame. I was hoping to provide suggested readings for pre-menstrual girls.

There were no comparable stories on the shelves or referenced in the librarians' resource materials. What was there reflected popular culture and focused on families and children with problems. There was no subtlety, no dignity.

Menstruation was more likely to be portrayed as an indignity, a curse even in adult literature and certainly an afterthought of life. Thus happening upon the dearth of sensitive materials for pre-menstrual girls determined the format for AHN'S STORY.

My original vision was:
Two beautifully bound, gently illustrated companion journals.
This is a text-only version in a single binding.
My gardener and nature lover's heart
imagines wonderful pictures of Ahn's surroundings.
Detailed and broad water colors
tucked around the edges of the story.
Also packets of scented herbal sachets
are slipped into the books.
Add an inspiring CD of music
intertwined with nature's best sound effects.
This is already a team effort with my
sister-in-law providing a rough edit
and her encouragement. To think of how you will make this journal
yours and broaden the meaning of Our Stories inspires me to dream
on..

This information and opportunity to tell your story is for an adult, a mother, aunt, teacher, grandmother. It begins with comments that may be of help in mentoring this crucial stage in a girl's life. It offers suggested readings and provides a place for the mentor to record her own menstrual experience. Hopefully you have already read AHN'S STORY and the materials for your young, female journalists which begins with a short introduction and AHN'S STORY and provides space for a young girl to record her own experience of the monumental changes in her body and soul.

One of the positive results to come from the emphasis on feminism during the baby-boom generation has been more sharing among women. Subjects that were taboo are more approachable, as more information becomes available. One of the negative spin-offs at the same time was the in-your-face sexuality portrayed by popular culture. The 21st century should have all the answers in this area of menarche, human sexuality and reproduction; but books like <u>Reviving Ophelia</u> written at the end of the 20th century by Mary Pipher tell us adolescent girls are confused by the messages. And we hear young girls suffer debilitating loss in confidence as they enter their reproductive years in our culture.

One missing element in most of our children's lives as they mature is any formal rite of passage from childhood into adulthood. As you complete the adult material, the information and suggestions may help to provide you, as a caring mother and/or mentor, with an informal vehicle for this missing stage in our maturation. This is only a stepping off place. Your own experience can be of more value than this little story of Ahn.

AHN'S STORY was a gift. I know I wrote it; but I had to search in my heart where exactly it came from and why. Upon returning to my parent's retirement home to live, I took frequent walks in the forest surrounding the house. One spot, a favorite of my mother's, spoke to me in a new way. Years of tiny, isolated musings about those who walked these woods before me flowed together into this brief story about a young girl named Ahn.

This time of creativity was a time of reflection for me over my life and my roles as granddaughter, daughter, wife, mother, and now grandmother. I got quieter, more prone than ever to seek solitude. Clocks and watches became ornaments, computers and telephones intrusions. The story surprised me, and I had a need to share it. I sent it to both of my sisters-in-law (one the mother of a pre-menstrual daughter). They both offered encouragement. I began searching for like stories, hoping to offer a list of helpful fiction to young, pre-menstrual girls. I recalled that I had spent those years devouring the fiction and biography shelves of our local library. There might be some who like me would use fiction to help flesh out their life views and emotional responses to maturation.

By providing pre-cultural, historical, and cross-cultural stories of young girls staged during the time of their first mense, I hope our young readers might find a soft, natural and positive way to help sort out what it means to be female on this planet.

But there were no stories to be found. There were non-fiction informative descriptions of what happens to their bodies in book and video form. AHN'S STORY became more of a surprise to me in its uniqueness. Popular culture is full of images from which young girls could model their approaches to living life fully in the feminine. My take is that most of these call for some material want to be fulfilled in order to successfully navigate this part of life. It might be the right hair color is needed, the right make-up, the right clothes, the right tattoo, the right body piercing, later the right car. The worst want given girls by our culture is a desire for the right body type. Very few images these girls see stress finding their center, finding themselves, finding peace and coming to grips with the ultimate questions (i.e.: Why we are here on Earth? How can we form our relationship with our planet? What do we truly need to do to avoid the drama/trauma portrayal of life in popular culture? What should our goals be as we enter the adult world?)

I did find some wonderful fictional descriptions of the rite of passage from child to adult, but only in books written for adults. The beginning chapters of two books stand out. Morgan Llewelyn's books Druids and Horse Goddess tell of a young male and a young female in early Celtic societies. We are given an appreciation for the wisdom of these cultures shown in the importance they placed on coming of age rituals.

Joseph Campbell in his works also emphasizes the wisdom found in earlier groups that recognize the relationship between the natural world and the female body. Campbell's videos require deep inquiry.

Judith Duerk in her <u>Circle of Stones</u>, <u>Woman's Journey to Herself</u> invites us to think:

"How might it have been different for you, if, on your first menstrual day, your mother had given you a bouquet of flowers and taken you to lunch, and then the two of you had gone to meet your father at the jeweler, where your ears were pierced, and your father bought you your first pair of earrings, and then you went with a few of your friends and your mother's friends to get your first lip colouring; and then you went for the first time to the Women's Lodge, to learn the wisdom of the women? How might your life be different?"

I have asked some friends to share about their experiences. These were women born in the mid 1940s.

"It was very much taboo to talk about in my family. My mother never told me anything to prepare me—most girls in her family had started very late (16-17) and I was eleven, so she probably thought she had lots of years before she had to face it, and by then most girls find out from peers. I scared my younger twin sisters because I did not know really what was going on. When my mom came home from work, she still did not discuss it with me, but had her sister (my aunt who is ten years older than me and had been one of the late ones) try to explain things to me. Needless to say, it felt shameful rather than a natural proud rite of passage for a normal girl."

Another friend fared better

"I guess I could sum it up in two words: Girl Scouts. My mom was the leader of my troop all through elementary school and somewhere around the fourth grade we got booklets, which were very informative and easy to understand. My mom wasn't one to talk about personal stuff and neither was it a help that I had an older sister who was pretty introverted at the time. So when my time came along, I wasn't surprised, and my mom acted like it was cause for celebration! I guess I felt like the information could have been handled in a more personal way than I experienced. So when my daughter was in third or fourth grade, I invited all the moms and girls in our Girl Scout Troop to a meeting.

It turned out to be a wonderful session with several moms telling stories that I am sure the girls will remember to this day. Tam-Brands (manufacturer of personal hygiene products) had a free video as well as printed materials that also helped us break the ice. I remember the meeting as a lot of fun, and it made us all feel that we were: 'women in this thing together.' "

My own experience screams of embarrassment

Waiting for my first period I was given enough preparation from my mother that it was expected. However, I guess I thought it would happen once and that would be it. Sometime later, sitting in my slide-in-desk-seat in 8th grade, I had that feeling that my then future mother-in-law's term "sinkin' spell." really fit. Most of you will know this feeling if you happen to be sitting still when your mense begins. I had a conversation with myself for the next half an hour before I asked to be excused. I wasn't sure how much I needed to be concerned. My teacher, Mrs. Marshall, followed me out into the hall and suggested I go immediately to the school nurse. They quickly doubled up and pinned my skirt over the spot and sent me walking home. I never wore that skirt again; and knew that I was the topic of conversation for my classmates. Years later, my husband volunteered that he had been told all about the incident though he was in a different class. A quote from Fruits and Candies magazine ca.1900 instructs: "Girls between 11 and 15 should be wisely instructed by their mothers or they will do foolish things that they will live to regret." This Victorian age advice is profound on all levels. This was quoted in Carol Padgett's book <u>Keeping Hearth & Home in Old Alabama.</u>

Another book that could offer much, especially if you are from a Judeo-Christian background, is <u>The Red Tent</u>. This is a marvelous retelling of an Old Testament story from a woman's point of view. And just as my friend helped her daughter and friends experience, "women in this thing together' so does this Jewish author give us the menstrual experience from another time and place. The violence and earthiness of these suggested readings may surprise you. But read then from Genesis starting about the 27th chapter, and you discover this has always been a gory story. We tell the version about Leah and Rachel and later Joseph saving his family, and we filter out the rest.

Girls who could benefit from reading AHN'S STORY are as young as 9 and 10. And my sense is they need a mentor, a mother, a teacher, an aunt, a grandmother to encourage them in the best learning from the story. If there were truly good examples of this type of story out there, the stories might stand alone. But a guiding and loving introduction to womanhood will help the young girl better appreciate and value her body. The physical, emotional and spiritual changes that will be part of her life the next few years have been negatively interpreted by our culture. (See Carol Gilligan's work in the sources.) The circle of women sharing and caring helps weave a safety net around these young girls and introduce them to the power of life that they hold in their bodies in positive ways.

After reading AHN'S STORY I hope you will sense, my primary interest of connecting the reader to the natural world comes through the strongest. Hopefully on reflection, the questions and the thoughts below may offer you a vehicle for delving deeply into the experience of menarche. If you take the time to write your own experience, it may bring life changes into perspective for you as well as your daughter or charge.

Some basic questions/conclusions come from this short journey back in time with Ahn. Hopefully sharing these concepts will add to this important time in your daughter's life.

The first question has to do with change. Do we try to make the world stop for our children in an attempt to give their lives a stable base? This may be a mistake. Life is only change. *Is accepting the constant of daily, periodic and seasonal change a healthy way to live life?*

Females live life differently than males. In our efforts to be equal with men we were sacrificing the innate value of being women. Thankfully the pendulum is swinging back from the unisex arena and hopefully it won't swing too far. *Does being female offer an opportunity to understand what living and loving on this earth is all about?*

While nothing stands still, there are natural rhythms and cycles that can help us flow with the current of change. Also, birth and death are both constants in human life. We can better introduce both as natural and awesome patterns to our children. *Can tuning into the rhythms of life and death give us a perspective for fuller lives and finding joy?*

If we hold a bigger viewpoint in our adult minds of how life works, we can pass on valuable life skills to our children with each loss they incur. Harvest time often involves the loss of plants that produce the harvest . *When experiencing the pain of loss and separation, can these become times for reflection as well as opportunities for appreciating the importance of all relationships?*

We are beginning to understand the strengths of various cultural approaches to life on earth. The eastern cultures that are less materialistic have brought healthy ways of exercising our minds and bodies. If you haven't experienced some of these traditions such as yoga, mindfulness of our breathing, awareness of our emotional fluctuations—this is a good time. What you learn about you will be able to teach. *Are learning to enjoy our bodies and seeking mindfulness (neutral observance of our emotions) good coping mechanisms for daily living?*

Faith journeys have begun to spring from the institutional observations back to nature where they began. Priming ourselves with readings by authors like Llywelyn forces us to absorb our inborn relationship to earth. Slowing down and taking time to sense the mystery all around us can keep us secure. *Can observing the sacred in places we see everyday and finding the spiritual within ourselves help ground us to weather the crises of living?*

This earth, these creatures, this universe, these bodies are so far beyond our understanding. With each insight science gains, more questions spew forth. We take so much for granted. *Does learning the cosmology of our universe, the story that artfully combines our present scientific knowledge of the environment and how it came to be with celebration and awe, give us a basis for finding peace?*

There are concepts coming to the fore of our culture, which enhance all of these questions. One is bio-regionalism. This encourages us to acknowledge and care for the natural region where we live, the particular types of hills and streams that surround us. Another concept that often escapes our science classes is the awareness of the planet as an organism itself. It is a gigantic leap to leave our WASPish idea that this earth was put here for us to use. But once we find this knowledge we can realize the truths found in indigenous peoples that proclaim the spirit of the earth as being viable.

You might want to read AHN'S STORY aloud to your daughter, a little at a time. Pondering over the questions presented above will give you places for stopping and discussing your own sense of living as a female on this planet in our time.

There are three books that I now consider crucial in helping a girl with this journey into and out of the child bearing years. I wasn't even aware of these books when this material was first put together. Kristi Meisenbach Boylan has written two small volumes that address a woman's journey from the spiritual perspective: Seven Sacred Rites of Menarche and Seven Sacred Rites of Menopause. Don't wait too late to read them both. The final book I want to recommend is not just for women, but it will help you benefit from journaling as a vehicle for growth. Christina Baldwin's Life's Companion, Journal Writing as a Spiritual Quest.

Self-publishing this small work as a very ordinary post-menopausal grandmother is an effort to encourage others to birth similar and better stories. More contributions to this unexplored, even taboo genre, will give our daughters and granddaughters more ways to understand the beauty and sacredness of the feminine life journey. There is always the question; "Am I opening Pandora's

Box?" I'm afraid the silence of our culture in this vital area has put our children in danger, and that knowledge passed on in loving and caring ways will better equip them to live on this Earth.

Examination of Sources

Baldwin, Christina Life's Companion, JournalWriting as a Spiritual Quest, Bantam Books, New York, 1991.
Enables reader to share the author's spiritual journey and facilitates the use of journaling for growth and understanding.

Barlow, Connie www.thegreatstory.org/GreatJourney "A Co-Creative Ritual of Gratitude and Commitment,"
   We do not know how to celebrate our incredible universe. This web page provides ways to combine scientific accuracy with human need to stand in awe and worship that which is greater than we are alone.

Berry, Thomas, Swimme, Brian, The Universe Story, Harper-Collins, 1992.
A cosmologist priest and scientist write a description of the universe as science understands its unfolding.

Blume, Judy is an author whose contemporary stories for juveniles touched previously taboo areas such as menstruation. However, none of her many books offer full blown, positive models for being a woman. Yes, God, It's Me, Margaret, Simon Shuster Reprint 2001, It's Not the End of the World, Here's to You, Rachel Robinson, Forever are some of the titles.

Bonvillain, Nancy, <u>Native American Medicine,</u> Chelsea House Publishers, Philadelphia, 1997

Native American medicine teaches that emotional and social well being are essential to physical health. "The body, the mind, the spirit, and the environment in which people live are all addressed with remedies that treat the living being as a total system made of many parts and in complete harmony with its environment." (p.77)

Boylan, Kristi Meisenbach, <u>The Seven Sacred Rites of Menarche, The Spiritual Journey of the Adolescent Girl</u> and <u>The Seven Sacred Rites of Menopause, The Spiritual Journey to the Wise Woman Years,</u> Santa Monica Press, 1991. Marvelous approaches to the feminine journey of life; both volumes pull from all of our strengths as the reproducers of life.

Diamant, Anita, <u>The Red Tent,</u> Picadore USA, NY 1997.

Jacob's daughter Dinah (Dee nah) is the voice that retells the story of the twelve tribes of Israel from the feminine. Powerful in its reality, probing in its assumptions, this book brings the Biblical story 180 degrees with its female perspective. The setting of her approach is the tent set aside for menstruating women which becomes the place of sharing and mentoring for younger women.

Duerk, Judith, <u>Circle of Stones, Woman's Journey to Herself,</u> Luramedia, San Diego, CA, 1989.

These brief reflections and probing questions may take your journey as a woman in directions you hadn't anticipated.

Fulghum, Robert, <u>From Beginning to End, The Rituals of Our Lives,</u> Villard Books, NY, 1995. Fulghum of <u>Everything I Know I Learned in</u>

Kindergarten fame discusses ritual in depth. He points out: "There are passages in one's personal, solitary, secret life that are no less momentous. Puberty and adolescence are filled with such occasions—all those times when you alone know that some irrevocable alteration has come to your existence. The Celebration comes in solitude, with no tangible evidence of change of status." (p. 22) "Rituals are often silent, solitary, and self-contained. The most powerful rites of passage are reflective," he states on the back cover.

These statements are true. However he is coming from an adult male perspective. Females are beings who thrive on relationship. In the female perspective, finding someone to share and help explain the rite of passage as monumental as the first menstrual period may help in the perilous crossing through the adolescent years and the understanding of a body that is tied so strongly to the earth's cycles.

Gilligan, Carol, Lyons, Nona P., Hamner, Trudy J., Editors, Making Connections, Harvard University Press, Cambridge, MA 1990.

This research study of adolescent girls adds powerful credence to the other works that are sending up red flags about female development in our culture (See Mary Pipher). In the chapter entitled "The Body Politic" by Catherine Steiner-Adair, pages 166-169 the problems faced by all girls are strongly and repeatedly underscored, though this chapter is about eating disorders. Adair states: "The processes of identity formation and body ownership seem to occur simultaneously for girls as a major catalyst for ego development."(167) One suggestion from psychology for adolescent females that she quotes was for young women to discount their emotional feelings during menarche as not really part of their true selves. (168) "Rather than help the girl relate to her body, own her body and live in her body in a creative way that honors the cyclical nature of women, this suggestion magnifies the pervasive cultural reaction to females, which teaches them to deny the validity and reality of who they are as young women." (168) Adair also points out that our society socializes girls to nurture and value relationships and then proceeds to devalue those who are not autonomous and independent (male traits)—a double bind...

Ikeda, Daisaku, <u>SOKA Education, A Buddhist Vision for Teachers, Students, and Parents,</u> Middleway Press, Santa Monica, CA 2001.

Ikeda's mentor was Josei Toda, whose mentor was Makiguchi, a contemporary of Thomas Dewey. The latter felt educators to be meaningful needed to encourage students to become global citizens. Both Dewey and Makiguchi felt that students needed to experience the complex relationship between people and the land, between nature and society. They would be able to better understand the wider world by learning from their local community. (105)

Levey, Joel, Levey, Michelle, <u>Living in Balance, A Dynamic Approach for Creating Harmony & Wholeness in a Chaotic World,</u> Conari Press, Berkeley, CA, 1998.

A primer that can correct the misplaced emphasis on materialism of the post World War II generations and their offspring. A pragmatic resource book for living that by its nature counters the problems discussed in this work on young girls.

Llywelyn, Morgan, <u>The Horse Goddess,</u> Tom Doherty Assoc., 1982 <u>Druids,</u> Ivy Books, NY, 1991.

This author uses her strong characters to offer philosophy for living that goes back eons in Celtic history and mythology. She accomplishes a lot in helping her audience understand Irish origins. But more importantly she is an historical novelist who gives her readers deep insight in human nature, early culture, and their connections to the earth. Too bad she doesn't also write for younger readers.

McKibben, Bill, <u>Hope, Human and Wild, True Stories of Living Lightly on the Earth,</u> Hungry Mind Press, 1997. McKibben points out the reforestation of the Adirondack Mountains can give us all hope. Previously he had written a book called <u>End of Nature.</u> Rebirth and renewal are forces of nature that sometimes humble humans.

Padgett, Carol, <u>Keeping Hearth and Home in Old Alabama</u>, Menasha Ridge Press, Birmingham, AL 2002. This charming compilation of Southern Victoriana is a fun read.

Peterson, Brenda, "Women in Nature", p. 160 OPRAH Magazine, July 2002.

Brenda Peterson writes from Baja, California while on assignment from National Geographic Books, her latest book <u>The Gray Whales' Mysterious Journey.</u>

"For me, returning to the wilderness is like discovering an inner true north that helps me navigate my life. Without this wild mentorship, I might lose my way."

Alexa is an adolescent taken on the trip by her parents to see the whales. After observing the diamond in Alexa's nose and the pink hair Peterson comments on the depth of Alexa's reaction to being in the wilderness. "At a time when most girls her age are falling into the confusing, feminine dilemma of self-doubt and shrinking to fit into high school society, Alexa is reaching out to a vastly diverse, natural world. The wild will hold and mirror her biggest dreams. Natural rhythms of tide or wind will center her and soothe her adolescent fear that she is out of place."

Pipher, Mary, <u>Reviving Ophelia, Saving the selves of Adolescent Girls,</u> A Grossett/Putname Book, New York, 1994.

An alert to the dangers built into our culture that are destroying the confidence and maturation of adolescent girls.

Stone, Jana, <u>Every Part of This Earth Is Sacred, Native American Voices in Praise of Nature,</u> Harper, San Francisco, 1993.

There are many environmentally sound and beautiful books and videos available to share with young women that emphasize a more basic way of viewing our earth.